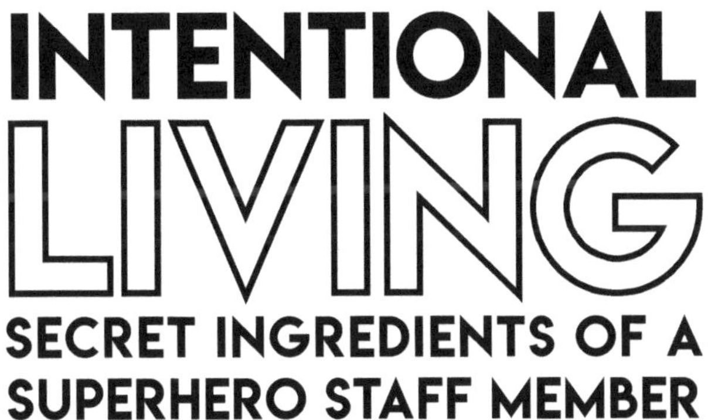

INTENTIONAL LIVING

SECRET INGREDIENTS OF A SUPERHERO STAFF MEMBER

AKSHAY DINAKAR

FOR
THE PADAWANS

SHOUTOUT TO THESE GOOFBALLS

ELLE BILLMAN
KAREN DAI
TIMOTHY LANN
JASON MCRUER

A LITTLE THOUGHT

There's no such thing as the "RA Personality." Being a successful RA isn't about being uber-extraverted, unbelievably creative, or flawless. No one is perfect, and it's dangerous to pretend to be.

Being a superhero RA is about self-reflectivity, knowing your strengths and limits, and having the commitment to instantly adapt to your environment.

There's no better position than an RA for becoming aware of your vulnerabilities and personal growth points, and catalyzing your development as a social leader.

Superhero staff members think deeply, and act fast. Learning as you go, re-framing problems as opportunities, and having a bias-towards action will take you far.

Building a community takes planning, effort, and most-importantly, **intention**. I metaphorically think of intention as the moral of a story – it's the holistic take-away or conceptual effort behind every event you organize, every conversation you have, every hug you give.

This book seeks to give you a starter-kit of intentions to experiment and play with. These aren't rules – they're simply ideas with potential. Make them your own, and have fun...

MY CONTEXT

Every Stanford University acceptance letter contains the following line:

"We look forward to your unique and extraordinary contributions to this campus."

Putting on a cultural psychology hat, it's evident that Stanford values an independent mindset in their students, and that's fantastic...but in the hustle to be the next famous individual, students often forget the underlying intention of college: to bring diverse and inspiring people together. We get so caught up in our own journeys that we undervalue the time we have with each other. It's true that college is a time to focus on yourself – but that's also how people burn out – it's important to find a balance, and my mission as an RA is to help others realize that.

As a product designer and psychologist, the best thing that happened to me at Stanford was the chance to staff Lantana, our "design-thinking dorm." All that term means to me is that we don't blindly repeat what's been done before – we prototype, we build, we empathize, and we create a truly innovative community that lasts far longer than the year that we live together in the same building.

They say that "where you live is the best reflection of who you are." This book is a collection of my personal actions and intentions that helped me transform Lantana from a house, into a home.

01

STYLE GUIDE

THOUGHT //

Branding is everything. Group culture is built around the symbolism of logos, teams unite behind a mascot, recognizable colors bring together people and places. Why are national flags considered so sacred?

INTENTION //

How might you create a culture through branding for your dorm? A style guide is a great way to dive in.

ACTION //

- Identify 3-5 words that define the culture you want to build. For Lantana, we chose "confident, creative, uplifting, cozy, and vibrant."
- Select a palette of colors and fonts that visually capture the sentiments of your culture words.
- Combine these elements to design a cohesive logo for your dorm. Put it proudly on your spirit wear, your emails, and defend its honor like a family crest.

02

SPIRIT WEAR

THOUGHT //
A good spirit wear design is one that people want to wear outside the dorm, not just inside it.

INTENTION //
Design spirit wear for the public eye, not just for the comfort of your residents.

ACTION //
- Consider spirit wear a physical artifact of your culture. Why do startups invest so much money and effort into the swag they give away at career fairs?
- Create designs that you would want to wear every day. If you're not excited to wear your own design, no one else is going to wear it, either.
- Having well-designed spirit items makes outsiders respect your dorm and the culture you have built. It's a great marketing tool of showing that your staff is on top of their game, as well.

03

FOOD

THOUGHT //
Consider presentation, interaction, and individuality when using food as a community-builder.

INTENTION //
Never order pizza. Choose food that allows for individual customization, engagement, and takes a while to eat.

ACTION //
- When deciding on what food to have at an event, consider the following factors:
	- What connects this food to the theme of the event?
	- How long does it take to eat this food, and what prevents someone from taking it and leaving without engaging in the event?
	- How can you design the layout/ presentation of the food, so that people hang around and socialize?
	- How can you make ordinary food feel/look fancy? College students love gourmet experiences.

04

BAKING

THOUGHT //
College kids love things that are fresh-outta-oven. Nothing feels more like home than some warm n' melty chocolate chip cookies.

INTENTION //
If you don't know how to bake, learn how.

ACTION //
- If you have the time, baking things is always better than buying them. It doesn't take that much skill, you improve your kitchen chops, and it tastes better than supermarket snacks.
- Baking treats allows you utilize the resources in the dorm, showing residents that you are physically engagedwith the space.
- It also sets a positive precendent for how other residents can use the dorm kitchen spaces for community-building.

05

RINGER

THOUGHT //
Get into a culture of talking with your residents over the phone, rather than texting. Talking feels personal, and you can chat fast without misunderstandings. If it's a sensitive topic, it's also nice to have it off-the-record.

INTENTION //
Choose a ringtone you like.

ACTION //
- Try to keep your ringer on as often as you can (except for class, duh).
- Experiment with sleeping with your ringer on. Depends on your level of nighttime dedication, but it has helped with some odd-hour crises before.

06

GROUP CHATS

THOUGHT //
The best group chats are defined by active participation, clear purpose, little-to-no spam, and rich visuals/media.

INTENTION //
Group chats are incredible community builders, if utilized correctly.

ACTION //
- If you're going to post a public announcement, be as concise and entertaining as possible. Use photos!
- Show your support by liking lots of messages, and encouraging others who are taking steps to build community.
- Before you post, ask yourself if you could DM a person instead of sending EVERYONE in the chat another notification.
- Make the purpose of the chat clear with the name/logo. When you first create the chat, send an uplifting post laying down some ground rules.
- Think about positive messaging. Every message you send should create at least two smiles - one for yourself and someone else.

CASE STUDY

THE NOOK

Keep an eye out for underutilized physical spaces, and re-design them to be spots for community building.

Lantana's third floor staircase had a strange alcove that had nice sunlight, but was uncomfortable and felt ambiguous.

Cut out some vinyl patterns, bought some fitting pillows, screwed in some floating bookshelves, and voila! The Nook was born.

Tip: Include a definition of your space that lays out a clear intention, so that residents know how to fully enjoy it!

Here's how we defined The Nook:

nook
/noun/
1. a small corner, alcove, or recess
2. a cozy place where you might open a new book, finish your pset, take an afternoon nap, and set your creative mind free.

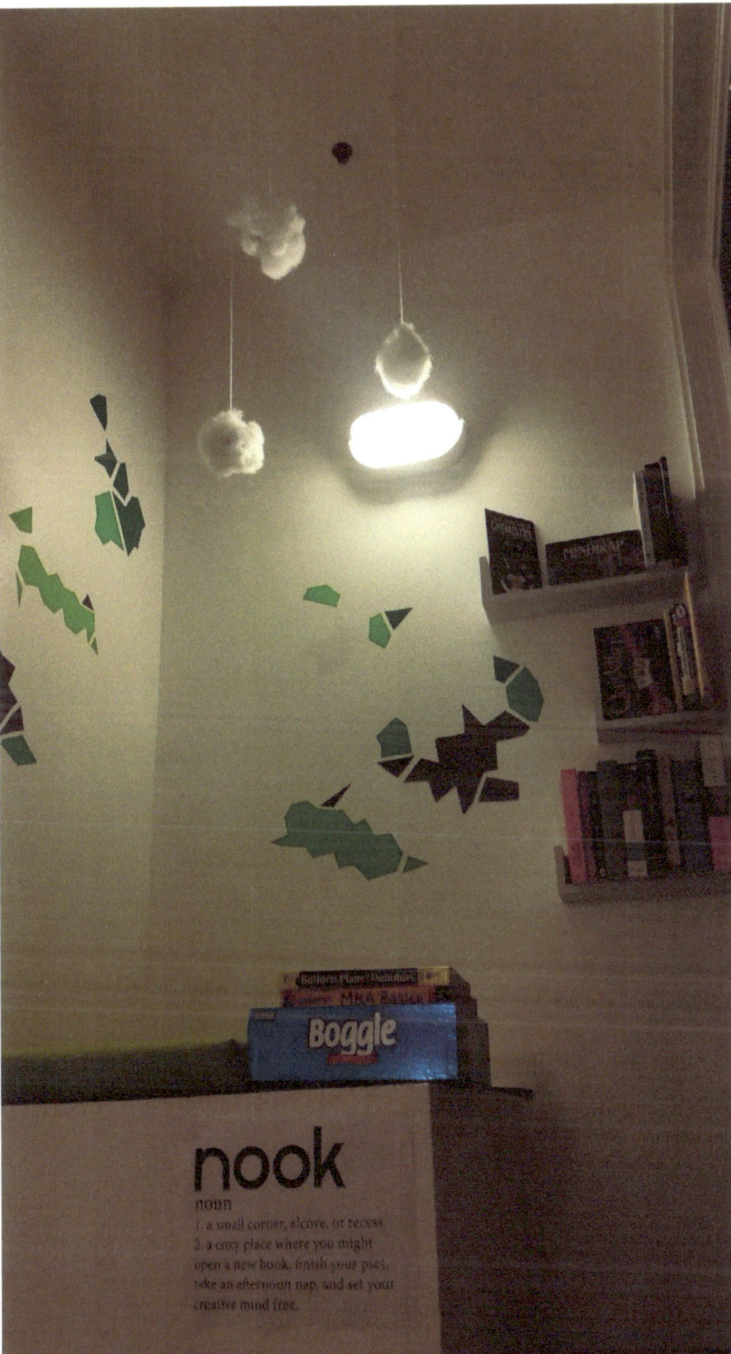
Boggle
nook
noun
1. a small corner, alcove, or recess.
2. a cozy place where you might
open a new book, finish your pset,
take an afternoon nap, and set your
creative mind free.

07

ARTIFACTS

THOUGHT //
Whether you're buying or building, design community items that are unique, represent your culture, and are multi-purpose.

INTENTION //
Fill your living spaces with interactive objects. We all love new toys.

ACTION //
- Design an item for your hall to use. Here are some things I built for my hall:
- Community Cube: a whiteboard cube that has candy and snacks hidden inside.
- Laser-cut acrylic keychains: help you identify your keys, while enhancing dorm branding.
- Indoor water fountain: creates a natural effect, and allows students to make wishes by putting good-luck coins inside of it!
- Wooden checkerboard (coins have residents' names on them).
- Self-driving mini-car + gondola robot that delivers snacks to the dorm.
- Interactive loveseat: forms an eclipse when your heartrate matches with a partner.

08

GOLDEN SIZE

THOUGHT //
Groups of 12-15 people are perfect for community building. It's just large enough where it's easy to make new friends (without folks hanging out in pre-existing cliques), and not small enough to where people feel uncomfortably intimate.

INTENTION //
Medium sized events are awesome for helping students make new friends. Capping an event at 15 people is not a bad idea.

ACTION //
- Design an event that would be perfect for 12 15 people. Include opportunities for new friendships to form as part of the experience.

09

BATHROOMS

THOUGHT //
Bathrooms are an underutilized common space for building community. It's arguably the only common space that every person enters each day, yet we don't maximize its potential.

INTENTION //
Prototype creative ways to spark conversations and make restrooms less awkward experiences.

ACTION //
- Re-think the purpose of common components of bathrooms. Shake things up, break patterns.
- Can a mirror be a post-it note wall with intriguing conversation starters, or self-care challenges? Can a stall door be an interactive piece of art, or message-board?

Example: In Lantana, a bathroom paper-towel dispenser's handle broke. Instead of contacting the housing staff, we decided to design and 3D-print our own, more ergonomic handle. It's now a conversation starter.

10

MOVE PEOPLE

THOUGHT //
When organizing off-campus adventures,
it's worth thinking about transportation, and
how the experience of traveling from point
A to point B can be as memorable as the
destinations.

INTENTION //
Consider the intention of your trip, and how
your mode of transportation can enhance it.

ACTION //
- Is getting a big bus the best way to
transport your dorm? How about a larger
number of smaller cars?
- Does your city have good public
transportation? Expose your residents to the
real world, and/or have a brunch party on a
train!
- Walking is not necessarily a bad thing,
especially if you are discovering your
destination as you move.
- Build in moments of spotaneity - let some
variables (such as which Uber residents take)
be random.

11
PERFECT EVENTS

THOUGHT //
How do you create consistently successful programming?

INTENTION //
Perfect events are not that hard to design, if you have the right ingredients.

ACTION //
- It's hard to make events exciting for others if you aren't excited about it yourself. Filter the events you choose to organize by first asking yourself, "Would I be willing to skip a final because this event is so darn cool?" Also, please go to your final.
- Perfect events have the following ingredients:
     - A low threshold of entry. They don't require a complex skill or narrow-scoped interest.
     - They have tangible takeaways – either physical items or photos/memories that participants walk away with.
     - They are worth telling a story about. Design experiences, not events – and as long as at least one person loves it, it's a success.

12

WORKSHOPS

THOUGHT //
Workshops are events where students have contagious fun while learning a practical skill. Emphasis on the contagious fun.

INTENTION //
Workshops are too often boring and ineffective, because they focus more on the learnings than the experience. It's possible to reverse this.

ACTION //
- Workshops can be highly successful dorm events if you choose the right skill to teach, and do it in a way that leads to lots of learning, without too much effort.
- Teach a skill that will have positive implications/direct impact, even after the event is over. Relevance is key.
- Two workshops we hosted in the dorm this year are Lantana Community Robots and Lantana Community Lamps, where students learned how to buid their own functional robots for the dorm, and customized nightlights for their doorways.

13

ACTION MEALS

THOUGHT //
How do you go about getting a meal with a resident you don't know very well, but want to help them/involve them more in the dorm?

INTENTION //
Action meals are a fantastic and productive way to get to know someone, and take actionable steps towards bringing them into the dorm.

ACTION //
- Rather than ambiguously/awkwardly asking someone to grab a meal with you, text them a clear itinerary of items you want to talk about.
- Make two of those items things that you know about them (extracurricular activities/ favorite hobbies) so that you can get to know them better, and make the third action item a way they can use their specific interests to get more involved in the dorm.
- Residents are always excited to team up with staff members to get involved in dorm life, but they might just need a little more confidence/guidance.

14

FLAKING

THOUGHT //
College students are kids pretending to be adults, and everyone unintentionally flakes at some point (some way too often).

INTENTION //
Be aware of flakiness, and organize your events accordingly so that you don't waste dorm funds.

ACTION //
- The Flakiness Factor (FF) is well-known. Though this number differs based on the cultural context of your college campus (flakiness is much more prominent on the West Coast than the Midwest), a good rule of thumb is that only 75% of the students who sign up for your trip will actually show up, even if your trip is as cool as flying to the moon.
- I fondly think of the Flakiness Factor as the "reliable statistic of unreliability."

CASE STUDY

SMOOTHIES

Midway through the school year, we won grant funding to buy our dorm a Vitamix smoothie machine – an item which has been incredibly effective at building community.

We presented it as a reward to our residents for keeping the kitchenette clean (studies suggest that positive reinforcement can change behavior, and is more effective in the long-run than negative reinforcement).

Smoothies are super easy to make, and are a manifestation of the idea that when joy is shared between people, it actually multiplies. Make one fill of smoothies, and 10 people can enjoy it.

It's become an easy-to-make (and relatively healthy) surprise treat for residents while studying, and a pre-game tradition for our dorm intramural teams.

Inspired by the success of the Vitamix, we just secured grant funding to get a dorm Espresso machine!

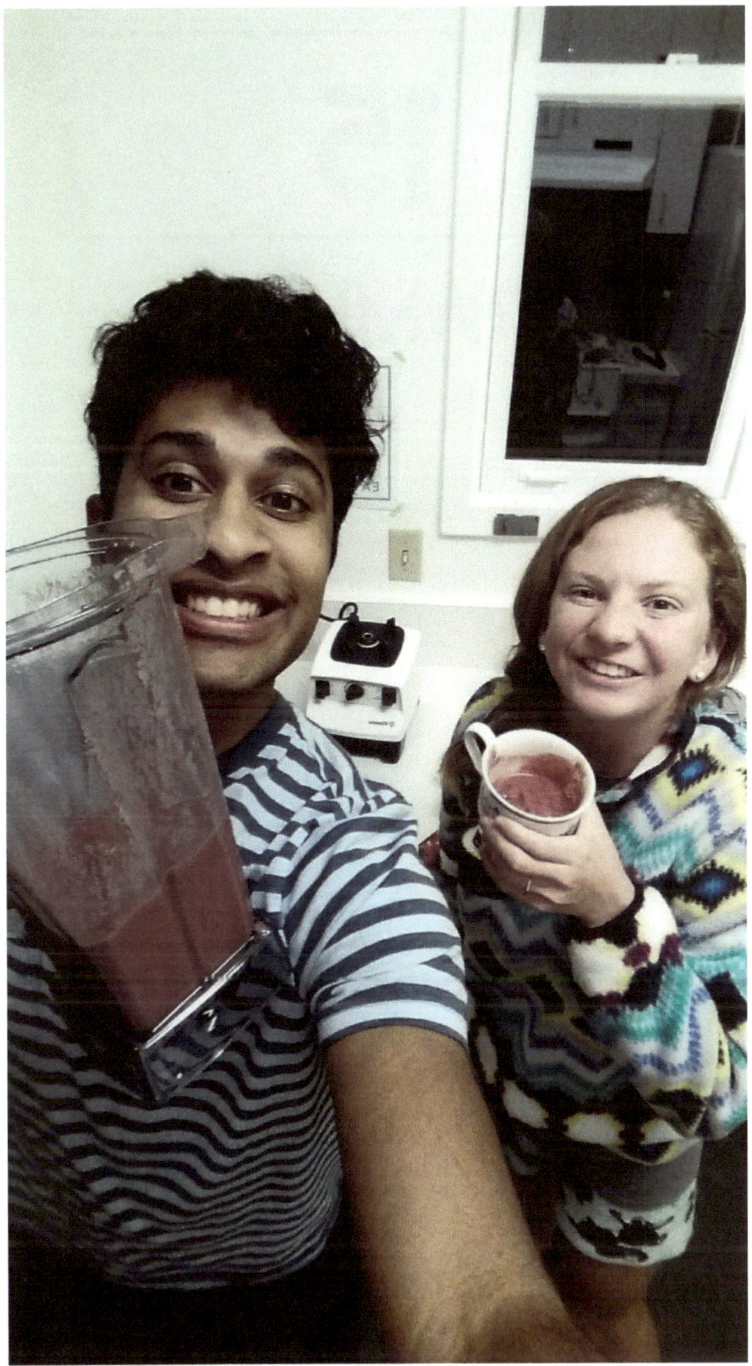

15

INTRAMURALS

THOUGHT //

Students sit in their rooms and study too much. How can you get students fresh air, and have regularly scheduled time for community bonding?

INTENTION //

Intramural sports are a great way to build dorm identity, keep your residents active, and learn how to work together for a common goal. Competing in different sports lets you attract various residents during the year.

ACTION //

- Dorm jerseys are great branding, and make your residents feel like athletic superstars. Have some fun with it – we had our own Lantana Media Day and did portrait shoots of all our intramural athletes.
- When coaching your intramural team, your first goal should be for your team to learn how to play together, and only after that – to focus on winning. Unconditionally support students who have joined your team, even if they aren't quite at Olympic level in the sport.
- Be respectful, uplifting, and get that win!

16

MINI-GAMES

THOUGHT //

How can you spice up life in a form factor that is playful and free-form (Unlike an event or trip, which has a set duration and is linearly structured)?

INTENTION //

Mini-games lead to laughter, higher engagement, and spontaneous moments of delight.

ACTION //

- Design mini-games with objectives that encourage students to break out of their daily routines, and engage with others/ physical spaces in the dorm. Motivate participation with prizes, if necessary.
- Here are some of my favorites:
    - Water gun Team Assassins.
    - Real-life Pokemon Go.
    - Hall Puzzles: Mystery balloons with resident fun facts, or word-search puzzles with resident names
    - Sneak a fruit into my dorm room without me noticing.
    - Impromptu pillow fight.

17

INTERACTIVITY

THOUGHT //
Home is an interactive environment. You can pin decorations onto walls; you can curl up on sofas; you can control your surroundings.

INTENTION //
Design your physical spaces for customizable interaction. Students love to touch, taste, smell, and look - and we all have varying levels of curiosity, and comfort preferences.

ACTION //
- Create a variety of ways to sit down. Where there are places to sit, people will spend time. Adapting your environment to the comfort of your guests is a key component of good hospitality. There's so many options for sitting down in my RA room – relax on my memory foam "friendship futon," chill in my circle lounge chair, sink into my bean bag, or plop down on my light-up cube.
- Whether it's vinyl stickers on walls, post-it notes, or portable chairs – choose furniture that move, and decorations that are meant to be touched.
- Design for impact, customizability, and durability.

18

REARRANGE

THOUGHT //
There's no such thing as the "optimal blueprint." Spaces need to be constantly adapted based on their current intended use.

INTENTION //
Staff members can broadcast that they care about their dorm by constantly rearranging the common space layouts. Side benefit – keeping things fresh makes your residents curious to engage with those spaces.

ACTION //
- Whenever you have an event in a common space, move around the furniture to better suit the purposes of your event. Environment adapts to you, not the other way around:
- Storytelling event? Drag the sofas closer, or have people sit on the floor.
- Arts/Crafts event? Think about the flow of people grabbing materials, snacks, and having ample table space to create.
- Before your event, envision the movement of your attendees, and tweak your space to subconsciously guide them to where you want.

19

AUTHENTICITY

THOUGHT //
Your mom's lunch-box notes. Hallmark cards. Phone calls. What makes them feel so heartwarming, and natural?

INTENTION //
Get off your computer, find an ink pen, and start handwriting notes.

ACTION //
- Handwritten items feel authentic – Times New Roman does not.
- Have a unique signature so that you can 'brand' your notes with your RA persona.
- Put some thought into what type of paper you write notes on.
- Write thank you cards/good luck notes to members of your community. It's a simple, self-paced way to stay in touch with residents you may not see that often. They'll often write back, resulting in an adorable local-pen-pal relationship.

20

ADAPTATION

THOUGHT //
When user testing a new product or solution, it's important to remember: it's never the user's fault. Everything can always be designed better.

INTENTION //
Take the time to learn who your residents are, and treat them the way they want to be treated.

ACTION //
- In the first few weeks of the school year, learn who your residents are. When are their birthdays? Favorite candy? When do they sleep? What's their cultural context, and what are their social goals in terms of dorm-life?

Cultural Psychology Tip:
Understand if your resident has more of an independent or interdependent mindset. This will help you effectively counsel them (if needed), give them social advice, and design experiences that they will be excited to participate in.

21

OUT-SOURCING

THOUGHT //
Be a CEO staff member. Craft a vision, an agenda, a game plan – and find others who are talented and excited to do the execution, so that you can focus on the creative leadership.

INTENTION //
Team up with residents who enjoy different types of tasks, so that they can support you in a way that they like!

ACTION //
- Something in the bathroom broke? Team up with a mechanical engineering resident to fix it.
- Want to host an arts/crafts event? Find the artists in your dorm and have them hop in the car with you to the paper store to choose the materials.
- Going to a nursery to buy plants for your hallway? Invite a student gardener to come with you to help educate your picks.

22

INCLUSIVITY

THOUGHT //
How does your persona, language, and appearance influence the degree to which residents feel safe/at home in the dorm?

INTENTION //
Educate yourself on diversity, and always be willing to engage with it, understanding that there are many ways to culturally "live life correctly."

ACTION //
- Visit all the cultural centers on your campus and familiarize yourself with their resources.
- Host cultural events in your dorm and have an open dialogue about diversity.
- Wear outfits that are respectful of other cultural groups.
- Think before you open your mouth. Then, think again before you make a sound.
- Follow the politics and movements of minority/oppressed groups. Learn how to develop opinions, but be a neutral facilitator when you need to be.
- Know and use your preferred gender pronouns.

RULEBREAKING

Your job as a staff member isn't to be a police officer. It's more appropriate to think of yourself as a supreme court judge – critically questioning the ethics of rules, and facilitating respectful obedience of them...as well as pushing for change when necessary.

There is much ambiguity in rules when running a dorm. It's like having a year-long sleepover with a 100 or so teens. You have no choice but to invent new rules and precedents on the fly.

I'm a firm believer that if a rule is broken in a respectful, uplifting, and intentional way that is fundamentally harmless but builds community, I am willing to re-evaluate my view on enforcing it. Here's an example.

Two residents on my floor were given a warning notice by the housing staff to move some boxes from the hall outside their door, or they would face a fine. Instead of trashing the boxes, they built a cardboard castle for the floor. All I did was move it to a more prominent spot – the alcove – simultaneously endorsing their creative thinking, and ensuring that their masterpiece wasn't a fire hazard.

HALL HANG

Coming into the school year, I was adamantly against hosting hall meetings. While a well-intentioned concept, the traditional hall meeting is mundane, inefficient at distributing information, and fails to achieve its essential goal of helping people in the hall become friends.

However...students continually expressed an interest in having some sort of regular hall gathering, so I decided to prototype the concept of a Hall Hang.

They say that humans (and especially the younger generations) have a 20 minute attention span – which is why TED talks are only 18 minutes long.

Hall Hangs are quick + unique gatherings that involve food and mini-games that reinforce collaboration, playfulness, relaxation, and a focus on interpersonal connection.

By focusing on designing a weekly experience that focuses on forging friendships rather than disseminating information, Hall Hangs are a highlight of my residents' week.

23

MUSIC

THOUGHT //
Everyone likes music. How might you utilize music and technology to build community?

INTENTION //
Use music as an common medium to engage diversity.

ACTION //
- Most music streaming services (Spotify, Soundcloud, YouTube, etc.) have a collaborative feature to them. Make your resident a collaborative playlist filled with artists you think they'll like – this is a great way to dive into a new friendship.
- Use a bluetooth speaker (at a reasonable volume) in the shower. One of my highlights was going to the gym with members of my floor, and then taking a "group shower" while blasting chill vibes when we all got back.
- Play music out loud, rather than using headphones. First, it's better for your ears. Secondly, having earbuds in makes people think you're either in-the-zone, or on a phone call – and it makes you less approachable.

24

ANNOYANCES

THOUGHT //
Whenever you bring a diverse set of people together, there will be little moments of conflict, and behavior of others that might irritate you.

INTENTION //
Understand why residents engage in those behaviors, and come up with creative opportunities to transform those annoyances into positive contributions to the community.

ACTION //
- Reframe the annoyance as a strength of that person's character, and combine it with an aspect of dorm life that will give that person confidence to use the annoyance in an uplifting manner.

Example: I had a group of boys who were notorious for kicking a soccer ball after quiet hours. I recruited them to our dorm intramural team – giving them added privileges like helping me create the jersey design. Their new level of involvement in the dorm gave them more respect for the community and they stopped the nighttime shenanigans.

25

IMMATURITY

THOUGHT //
College kids are lucky in that they don't have the burden of being full adults quite yet – make sure your residents don't forget that.

INTENTION //
Help your residents loosen out, relax, and remember that they don't have to be so serious all the time.

ACTION //
- Have a interesting wardrobe. Really consider what clothes you wear, and don't be ashamed to put on silly outfits to lighten the mood, especially around midterms-time. Ever since losing a bet freshman year, I've been required to wear a Lemur onesie to brunch every Sunday morning, which causes all sorts of giggles.
- I'm always pranking my residents and goofing around. Whether it's a Nerf Gun sneak attack, spraying students with Silly String, or teaming up with their roommates to scare them, make sure your residents are laughing every day.

26
OTHER DORMS

THOUGHT //
How might you make your dorm feel like THE place to live, while still being respectful of and collaborative with other dorm communities?

INTENTION //
Rather than assert your dorm as the most superior residence, think of your dorm as a role model community that exists to inspire other nearby residences.

ACTION //
- Make friends with the staff members of other dorms, and have an open dialogue with them. Share the trips you're going on, give them copies of your grant applications, and team up with them for select events.
- Welcome students from other dorms into yours as visitors. For the external students who are hanging out in your dorm all the time – make them honorary residents! Having a thriving dorm "tourist industry" makes your residence a "elite" place to live, and visitors bring a lot of fresh energy into your community.

27

INTRIGUE

THOUGHT //
How might you create a sense of positive intrigue in your dorm that inspires a social curiosity in your residents?

INTENTION //
Learn how to keep secrets, be mysterious, and make lots of physical interventions without initial explanation.

ACTION //
- Repurpose ordinary objects. Blow up a balloon, and hang it from the ceiling like a chandelier.
- Make subtle, unexplained changes. Move a table from one side of a room to another.
- Hide lots of things. Especially effective if there's a pattern to the hidden items (this was the main idea behind real-life pokemon go).
- Drop lots of clues, both physical and digital. Plant lots of 'Easter Eggs' in your emails, and use foreshadowing in the physical wall-decorations.
- Use red herrings to throw off the residents who are hot on your trail!

28
SPONTANEITY

THOUGHT //
How might you inspire your residents to live more vibrantly, creatively, and organically?

INTENTION //
Create heartwarming surprises.

ACTION //
- Tape surprise good-luck notes, puzzles, and doodles to your residents' door handles (this is the most effective place to put something that you want seen).
- Go analog. Be physical instead of digital. Example: replace digital Google forms with doodle polls made out of giant scraps of paper on the walls of your staircases.
- Be high-energy, and high-action. Throw candy at your residents. Engage them at unexpected times (whenever I get midnight snacks for my residents, we call it a "Hall-nighter"). Give lots of hugs and high-fives. Create secret handshakes.
- I like to sometimes go temporarily "incognito": I disappear from the dorm for a day and reappear with some sort of delightful new intervention.

MYSTERY TRIPS

Mystery trips are well-designed off-campus adventures that are filled with intrigue, center around unique experiences that catalyze friendships, and are delightfully unforgettable for everyone involved.

We launched Mystery Trips as a concept midway through the year. A limited number of residents can sign up for select spots, knowing just a few clues about their potential destination. They hop in a car, and we drive off and have a great time, whether it's ice skating, sunset hiking, pop-up concerts, or making homemade pizzas.

A tutti-frutti of intrigue, spontaneity, and breaking patterns, Mystery Trips have been some of the community building highlights of our year in Lantana, and we hope to establish them as a tradition for years to come.

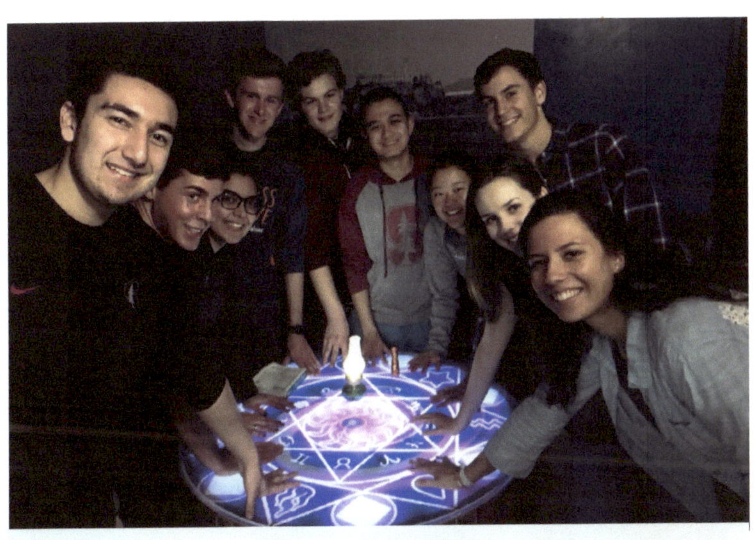

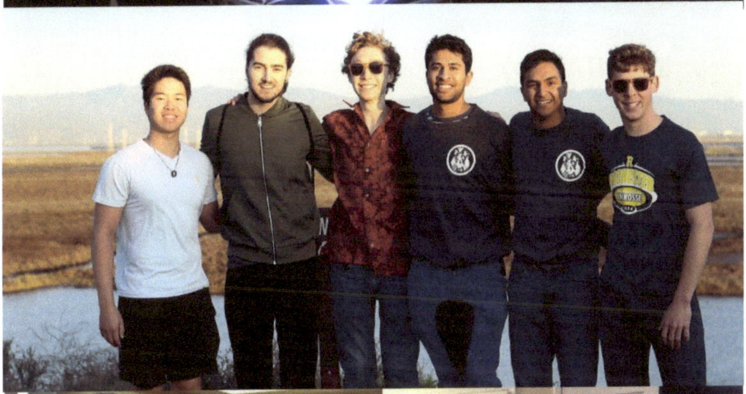

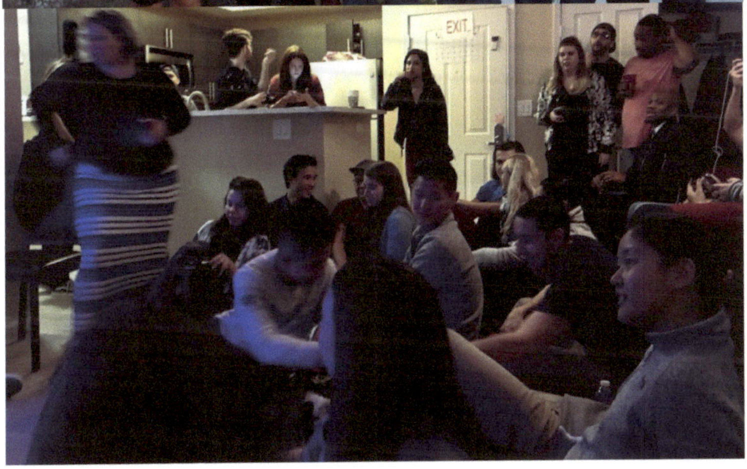

29

PRESENCE

THOUGHT //
How do you integrate RA-ing into your daily routine?

INTENTION //
Don't multitask. Instead, do tasks that serve multiple purposes.

ACTION //
- If you are walking from the first floor to the third floor, bring a bag of candy with you, and make sure it's empty by the time you reach the top floor.
- Create your own "conversation starter kit": a bag of treats and mystery items that random residents can reach into and grab, trying to guess what individual objects are. Reveal the object and tell the resident the story behind it, sparking a unique conversation.
- Consider your RA room the 'hotel lobby' of the floor. Learn how to keep a cozy and clean space, as if it's a five star hotel. High engagement, diverse function, and fantastic maintenance should define your space. Keep that door open – you never know who might just walk in and make your day!

30

WIN-WIN CONVOS

THOUGHT //
When you're dealing with conflict or ethical decisions, how might you achieve a happy outcome?

INTENTION //
Though it takes confidence and compromise, push yourself to achieve win-win outcomes in conversations with residents.

ACTION //
- When you're serving as the judge of a dorm mini-game, or forced to make an ethical decision, the easiest path forward usually involves favoring one party (the winner) and identifying another (the loser). As an RA, it's your job to help students work together to maturely discuss, debrief, and achieve a win-win outcome of a conversation.

Example: When regulating our dorm Assassins tournament, two teams were involved in a controversial ruling. I facilitated a conversation that resulted in both teams achieving a win-win resolution, and actually hugging each other after the win-win convo!

31

PLANTS

THOUGHT //
How can you make your environment feel more alive, healthy, actively loved, and natural?

INTENTION //
Consider the role of plants in your physical space, and how you can use them as a marketing tool to show that you care about your dorm.

ACTION //
- Plants make people happy. Decorate your common spaces with plants, and give them personality.
- Name your plants creatively. We named our plants after famous bossa nova musical artists, and challenged our residents to figure out the pattern in the plants.
- Teach your community to care about the plants. Come up with a creative way to get your community to water the plants, and treat them with respects. The Stanford design school made Twitter accounts for their plants, and had them tweet once a week: "I'm thirsty!"

32

PICTURES

THOUGHT //
How might you immortalize experiences, and vicariously allow those who missed out to still feel like a part of it?

INTENTION //
Take lots of pictures of dorm life, and document all that you've done. You can never take too many pictures in college.

ACTION //
- If you've got some photography chops, volunteer at the beginning of the year to take free portrait photos of your residents. This will allow you to quickly associate names with faces, and they'll feel grateful to you for taking free photos of them. That portrait photo is a start to your friendship with those residents, and every time they see that photo, they'll think of you.
- Use photos to create branding for your dorm. Capture memories. Print large posters. Insert photos into emails, GroupChats, and TV screens. Think about the presentation of a photo and how it influences the interaction of a viewer with the image.

33

EMAILS

THOUGHT //
What makes someone open, read, and respond to an email?

INTENTION //
People only open emails that they would want to respond to. Design your emails with a specific reader and intended response action in mind.

ACTION //
- The main idea: emails that lots of effort have been put into will be opened. Whether that's entertaining language, beautiful graphics, or concise messaging, those are the factors that attract engagement.
- Use a mixture of case letters in your subject line. ALL CAPS is overused, and all lowercase feels lazy and too informal.
- Don't use GIFs. They imply laziness, as someone has created the graphics for you. Integrating emojis can be effective.
- Use a precise color scheme (base this off of your style guide!) of just a few contrasting colors. DON'T simply use a full rainbow - it's overwhelming.

34

DOORS

THOUGHT //
Open doors build community. But how does one motivate others to keep their doors open?

INTENTION //
Shift in-room activity into the hallways, and creatively maximize the community-building potential of closed doors.

ACTION //
- Have surprise snacks in the hallway, and create whiteboards so that it is more comfortable for students to study in the hallway than inside their rooms. Moving activity to the hallways will result in people running out into the hall and leaving their doors open.
- Knock on doors when you get back to the dorm. Chat with the residents, and subtly leave the door open when you leave – students are too lazy to close the door and it will likely stay open. Open doors lead to more doors opening on their own.
- Tape puzzles, whiteboards, and doodle scraps to the outsides of closed doors, so engagement can still happen when they're closed.

QUIET HOURS

It's always been hard to motivate myself to enforce quiet hours. A firm believer that many of the best memories, conversations and adventures of college happen in the odd hours of the night, it's hard for me to command students to be quiet after 11 pm.

Not all students share this interpretation, and due to rigorous schedules, sleep early. The late night community thinks of them as the "complainers," but they're also the early-birds who are on top of their lives. How do we strike a balance between the two types of residents, without causing uncomfortable or frustrated nighttime interactions or passive-aggressive text messages?

There are several folds to this. First, empathy solves this problem – not text messages.

If you're making a lot of noise, chances are, you're not looking at your phone – so the text message is useless. Secondly, all the text message is going to do is make you feel angry at the "complainer" for being so 'lame' or 'antisocial.'

From the complainer's side of the equation,
they just want some sleep, and are often
too tired or shy to step out of their room
and have a face-to-face confrontation with
the noise culprits, since they might be more
dominant personalities.

Every dorm faces the quiet-hours-challenge,
and I decided to take a stab at solving
it. Inspired by hotel do-not-disturb signs, I
created cute, recognizable door handle signs
that say "I'm snoozing!"

This subtle cue alerts noisy nighttime folk that
someone is sleeping inside the room, and that
they should probably take their conversation
to a better location. It avoids the awkward
confrontation, and builds empathy between
residents as they learn what time their
neighbors go to sleep.

One of the most effective interventions of the
year, the "I'm snoozing!" door handle signs
seem to have entirely solved the problem.

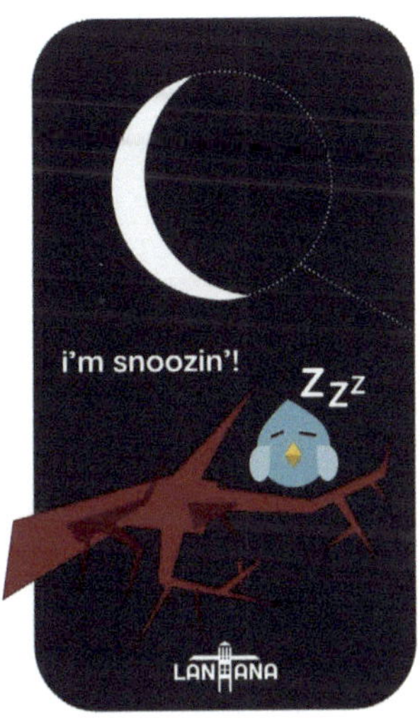

35

+ PSYCH

THOUGHT //
How do you craft your thoughts and statements to uplift others?

INTENTION //
As a social leader, the language you use makes an emotional impact on those around you.

ACTION //
- Never say "No" or "But." Get into the habit of saying "Yes", "And", "Absolutely," and "Sure." Even if you disagree with something, find a way to agree with part of it before you offer your counter-opinion.
- Be careful about making promises you can't keep, but encourage ideas from your residents, even if you're not completely on board. Work with your residents to critically think through their thoughts.
- Have unconditional love for your residents, and even if they do something that hurts you, make the honest effort to understand their intentions. They're your family – you can't reject or ignore them – learn how to live with them and bring out their best.

36
BETS & DARES

THOUGHT //
Students are too often scared of their staff members, or feel that they are unapproachable because they are too professional or intimidating.

INTENTION //
The best leaders know how to make a fool out of themselves, and embrace the fun of it.

ACTION //
- Make bets and dares with your residents. Make sure that you're the one who usually has to do the punishment, and ensure that they're never in an uncomfortable power dynamic, where they feel forced to do something uncomfortable.
- Your credibility and residents' respect for you will actually increase if you have the confidence to be a goofball.
- Experiential experiences result in higher satisfaction than material purchases. Consider this when designing the bets and dares you participate in.

SHOWER HAIR

Bathrooms (especially ones that aren't well designed) can get dirty. Oftentimes, it's a visitor to the dorm who messes up a common space (since they don't feel accountable/attached to the community) – so you should be careful to scold your residents before you've first figured out who created the mess.

A recurring problem in many women's bathrooms is shower hair not being cleaned up. I thought that it'd be an interesting design challenge to tackle.

After chatting with some women on my floor and scouting out the bathroom, I came to this hypothesis – shower hair is left on the floor of the bathroom because the effort required to clean it up is too high (one must pick up the hair with a paper towel and carry it across the entire bathroom to a trash can).

Sometimes, the simplest solutions are the best. I bought a trashcan and placed it right next to the showers. Problem solved.

Minimizing the threshold of effort for a unpleasant task makes it more likely that students will actually complete it.

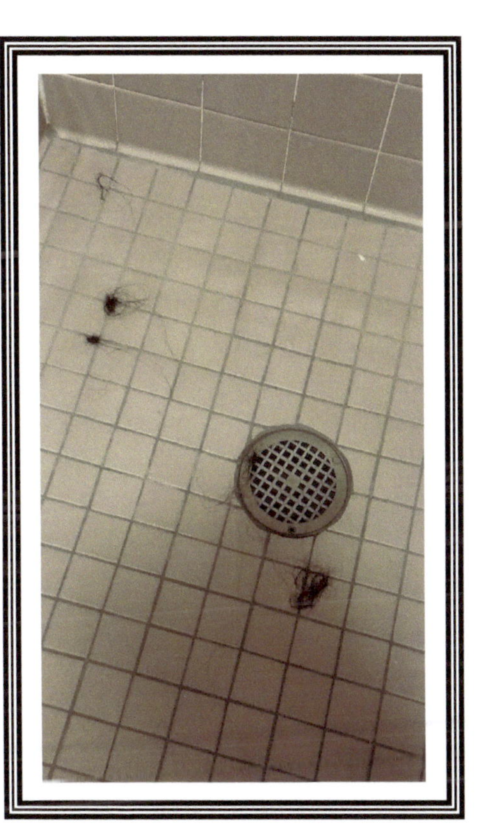

37

HARD CONVOS

THOUGHT //
Whether it's a crisis, enforcing rules, or distributing non-positive information, how do you dive into a difficult conversation with a resident?

INTENTION //
Have confidence, open-information, faith in your ethics, a bias towards action, and be thorough.

ACTION //
- The longer you put off a difficult conversation, the harder it will be and the more it will weigh you down.
- Be open. If you are honest and as matter-of-fact as possible, the resident will only have feelings against the situation, not you.
- Imagine the different directions that the conversation could go, and have a game plan for each. Craft the conversation towards a specific outcome, so that both you and the resident know what steps to take.
- Don't doubt your ability. Knock on that door and help the resident. You're doing the right thing.

38

TRADITIONS

THOUGHT //
Inventing your way forward means that you're setting the precedents and traditions for the years to come.

INTENTION //
Rituals are fun, symbolic, meaningful, and connect communities over time.

ACTION //
- Whether it's a theme song, a dorm flag, or a dialect that everyone recognizes, create some rituals that are manifestations of your dorm culture, with the intention of having these exist for many years.
- Traditions repeat themselves, which make them different from events.
  Traditions are patterns, not processes. Patterns can evolve and iterate over time, but incorporate the same motifs. Processes are step-by-step instructions that lack creative flexibility.

39

IMPERFECTION

THOUGHT //
Your greatest strength is not being perfect.

INTENTION //
Don't pretend to be perfect, but chase perfection.

ACTION //
- None of your residents want you to be perfect. Perfect people don't exist, and we don't know how to relate to them. They're lonely, and impossible.
 - Learn from your mistakes, and constantly prototype your way forward. Iterate, test, iterate. Keep track of your progress and be sure to celebrate the successes, large and small.
- Significance isn't about magnitude – it's about internal satisfaction. Though being a staff member is a very selfless job, remember that deep down, you're doing it for yourself. Smile when you feel proud of your work, enjoy the little moments, and most of all – love yourself for who you are and who you want to be.

www.ingramcontent.com/pod-product-compliance
Lightning Source LLC
Chambersburg PA
CBHW040232240726
48664CB00001B/99